Good-Bye, Incurable Diseases!

Kimihiko Okazaki, M.D.

iUniverse, Inc.
Bloomington

Good-Bye, Incurable Diseases!

Copyright © 2010, 2011 Kimihiko Okazaki, M.D.

The information, ideas, and suggestions in this book are not intended as a substitute for professional medical advice. Before following any suggestions contained in this book, you should consult your personal physician. Neither the author nor the publisher shall be liable or responsible for any loss or damage allegedly arising as a consequence of your use or application of any information or suggestions in this book.

iUniverse books may be ordered through booksellers or by contacting:

iUniverse
1663 Liberty Drive
Bloomington, IN 47403
www.iuniverse.com
1-800-Authors (1-800-288-4677)

ISBN: 978-1-4620-0428-7 (sc)
ISBN: 978-1-4620-0429-4 (hc)
ISBN: 978-1-4620-0430-0 (ebk)

Library of Congress Control Number: 2011903804

Printed in the United States of America

iUniverse rev. date: 10/22/2011

Contents

Preface

My hobby used to be constructing and fixing radios and record players. After graduating from high school, I took the entrance exam for a faculty of electric engineering and beautifully failed. During the extra year preparing for the next chance, I thought, *It would be much more fun to fix human illnesses.* I made up my mind to enter the faculty of medicine.

Graduating from the Kyoto University Faculty of Medicine, I had to enter a department after a year of internship. I chose fundamental medicine, accepting the invitation to a position of a university assistant.

In the second year of my tenure as university assistant, the professor gave me a research assignment. I was able to solve a problem that the teaching staff was unable to solve. In addition, I was so fortunate that I discovered a novel fact unexpectedly. As a matter of course, I expected to be evaluated. On the contrary, the professor told me to stop working on the discovery. Presumably he was afraid that the discovery would leak out.

I was displeased and quit the university assistant position, opting to enter the department of medical chemistry as a graduate student.

Afterward, the professor of medical chemistry gave me an opportunity to go to the University of Pittsburgh to work as a postdoctoral research fellow. I joined the laboratory of an assistant professor of physiology, who was an endocrinologist, at the University of Pittsburgh School of Medicine.

I succeeded in the project that the assistant professor gave me. On the basis of my success, he became the chairman of the biochemistry department at the University of Melbourne School of Medicine.

I wanted to stay in the United States for a while longer, and when I was introduced to a professor of microbiology, I entered his laboratory. The professor gave me a research problem, and I again succeeded in obtaining results that were worth reporting; the professor wrote an article out of my results. I then entered my third laboratory in the same school. The work I did in the third lab was published in *The Journal of Biological Chemistry*, one of the most authoritative biochemical journals.

Afterward I returned to Japan. I was invited to the department that I had left in 1963. I reentered there and resumed working on the problem that had been prohibited in 1962. After getting results and publishing them in *Biochemical and Biophysical Research Communications*, I was recommended to the position of assistant professor at Aichi Medical College, and I took the position in 1974.

Introduction

Although contemporary medicine seems to have made remarkable progress, it is still far from the state of controlling all diseases. Rather, many diseases are incurable by means of contemporary medical techniques.

For example, the principal trend in cancer treatment is to extirpate the tumor as early as possible. A surgical removal of sick organs cannot be regarded as a complete cure because the patient loses normal organs even though his life is saved temporarily.

In cases when it is too late, surgical treatments are contraindicated. Antitumor agents or radiation are applied instead, which may hurt normal cells, too. Consequently, the patient's physical strength is weakened and the life span is shortened. Therefore these treatments are not healing treatments.

Why has an epoch-making treatment for cancer not been discovered when the number of cancer patients has grown so large? Regarding treatment of hypertension, antipressure agents may reduce the high blood pressure, but the pressure would increase upon stopping the medicine. These treatments are not radical ones.

For another example, there is diabetes mellitus. Overnourished people tend to suffer from diabetes mellitus, and their number is rapidly increasing. The number of latent patients without any subjective symptoms is said to exceed thirty million in Japan. Patients of diabetes mellitus are treated by prescription of medicines that may control the levels of blood sugar and glycosylated hemoglobin, and so it may seem that the disease has healed. However, no radical treatment has been given, and the patients' physical conditions gradually worsen, for example, atherosclerosis as a complication of diabetes mellitus proceeds. In order to cure diabetes mellitus radically, restriction of food intake and augmentation of physical exercise are the only methods available today. Therefore, patients' personal efforts are essential.

The topics that I am going to present here are wonderful news for those who are suffering from collagen diseases that are regarded as incurable, from cancers, or from allergic diseases, for neither of which radical cure is yet established. Luckily, now, the above-mentioned diseases are no longer incurable but are completely curable.

This book will contain splendid information for those who have dealt with the diseases for a long time and have kept receiving treatments that were not very effective. You will be released from the diseases at last and resume peaceful lives sooner or later. Many of those who have obtained this book must be expecting that his or her incurable disease will heal completely. To serve these readers, the radical treatment is described in detail in chapter 1, with chapters 2 and 3 describing radical treatments of cancers and of diseases due to overnourishment, respectively.

In chapter four, problem of mind is discussed, although it is not directly related to the diseases with which this book deals. You may take a look at it after you have recovered from your disease, and I believe that you will acquire something from my information.

In chapter 5, I summarize my long-held ideas about the desirable features of global inhabitants. In the cosmos, there are innumerable stars in almost infinite space. There also are numerous planets on which highly civilized humanoid beings inhabit. It is not true that the earth is the only planet where highly intellectual species exist. It is just like the Ptolemaic theory of the Middle Ages.

As a matter of fact, many people seem to believe that the earth is the most highly evolved planet in the whole universe, but is that really so? This belief is merely a consequence of watching films in which space-men wars are shown, indicating alien inferiority.

In several places on the earth, a vast sum of money is consumed to arm their countries with nuclear and other weapons. Although many people are so starved that they don't know if they can survive the day, others stay in luxurious hotels that cost more than ten thousand dollars per night. The earning differentials are extraordinary. Why can't they be made more equal?

A few countries spend enormous parts of their national budgets for wars and armaments without spending taxes to relieve the weak and poor. These countries utilize advanced science and technology to develop weapons for massacre. I would like to ask statesmen and soldiers of such countries, "Which country on earth do you intend to use these weapons against?"

Why do they hold summit conferences so frequently? Isn't it to meet face-to-face, exchange words, and attain better understandings of each other's country? From where does the necessity of war against each other country on the earth come?

On other inhabited planets, alien beings must have completed their era of settling troubles and disputes by means of war a long time ago. On reflection, most human beings are as ignorant as a frog in the well, struggle against hard life, and finish their life spans without any great progress.

Apart from Japan, who has a peace constitution, even today there are people who get drafted, sent to war, and killed violently. Suicide bombers keep appearing; it is now a daily event that many people are involved in the bombings and die. This is the present global condition. It cannot be left as it is.

I wish to think about the future's global society with you through this book.

CHAPTER 1:
How to Cure Allergic and Collagen Diseases

Subsection 1: Contemporary People and Medicine Are Deeply Attached to Money

I believe that you would like to receive without delay a treatment that is good for allergic and collagen diseases if such a treatment was available. I also believe that you want to know where to go in order to receive the treatment. This book will give you all that information.

Please read this book to the end because allergic and collagen diseases, which used to be incurable, will heal completely without fail.

Most, if not all, readers think that scholars and doctors in the field of medicine make efforts to find causes of diseases and discover how to heal them. It is a matter of course to think that a novel therapy would spread all over the world promptly after the discovery, and patients of the disease would enjoy its benefit. However, this is not so.

A normal way of thinking is that the doctor wants to serve many people with the truth that has been discovered through his or her earnest research. But something is going wrong because our way of living has changed.

What do you think is the most important thing for most people? Sick people may say, "It's health." But what a great majority of people desire is money. For them, the purpose of life is to become rich. They simply think that rich men can do whatever they want and can spend a happy life without any worries.

Most people try hard to take as high a position as possible or to become famous either as athletes or in another field. Most parents expect their children to earn a good living.

The supreme aim of enterprises is to pursue gains. Employees who can contribute to this aim are regarded as capable and receive better wages. Employees of low efficiency are treated coldly and are released when the company struggles.

That is the case with hospitals, too. After purchasing modern equipment, the invested capital must be refunded as soon as possible. The means to obtaining that money is to make the patients pay.

I don't know if you notice it, but when you visit a hospital while your condition is not too good, hospitals often let you receive more than the necessary examinations, such as X-rays, CTs, MRIs, and the like. Some of you may have thought, *Won't just one exam do?* But hospitals have their own reasons and motivations. Examinations are carried out according to manuals and often require no special knowledge. Consequently, various examinations are indispensable financial resources for the hospital.

On the other hand, from the patients' viewpoint, their physical strengths are exhausted during many examinations, and their remaining life spans may shorten.

The story does not end with examinations. Many hospitals hold seminars to study how to stabilize their management. We would rather think that they keep studying days and nights for how to help patients and how to cure diseases completely. The reality is quite different.

The number of people who undergo blood dialysis is increasing. This is because the hospital wants to maintain a certain number of dialysis patients in order to bring about a stable income. It is time-consuming and unpleasant to undergo blood dialysis for the patient, but for the hospital, such patients are very welcome. Dishonest physicians are sometimes socially prosecuted because they intentionally treat patients in order to make new recipients of blood dialysis.

How about doctors who don't work in hospitals? A few doctors go to a remote place, open up a clinic, and support the health of the people of the area. They must be looked up to as wonderful persons. But most physicians consider their own situation first. Although we cannot blame only doctors because many contemporary people have forgotten the spirit of public service. Most researchers have strong desires for discoveries of novel treatments and for fame, and so they naturally oppose discoveries made by somebody else.

There is a similar circumstance in my own background. For some reason, my current method of practice meets a persistent resistance and won't spread into the world. This is the reason why I decided to write this book—in order to let you know directly about my method, which is capable of saving all of the approximately two hundred million patients of collagen diseases on this planet.

Under these circumstances, it is not guaranteed that you can receive the treatment at any clinic, simply because it is not widely known. Herein lies the problem.

What a patient expects and desires most is nothing but a complete cure of his disease. However, it is not desirable for the contemporary medical world to heal diseases easily that used to be incurable.

Subsection 2: Reasons Why Previously Incurable Diseases Are Not Cured Easily

Because patients incorrectly believe that collagen and allergic diseases are incurable, no one complains if an ineffective treatment is given for a long time. Hospitals want patients' money in order to keep running. Therefore it is desirable for hospitals to keep treating the resigned patients in the customary way. Medical centers would be unable to raise much money if an amazing discovery diffuses to the whole world, and those diseases are cured easily. If hospitals cannot raise money, they would be bankrupt. I don't say that all hospitals are like this, but unfortunately, these money-obsessed hospitals are gaining in number.

There are numerous circumstances in the contemporary medical world where the medical staff can profit. A considerable number of scholars study "incurable" diseases. Each scholar has his or her own research project and makes efforts days and nights. For them, a momentous discovery would be nothing but a nuisance—because their research would end and their funding would stop.

The method that I'm going to demonstrate in this book is extremely simple and clear-cut. It is so simple that few, if any, scholars would like to admit it. They must feel that their research field is being invaded.

However, as far as the patients are concerned, the research funding doesn't matter at all—what matters is whether or not the diseases are healed. It is utterly a matter of course.

The reason why I dare publish this book is only because I cannot help doing something for the patients. No matter what authoritative doctors say, what matters is whether or not the diseases heal.

Subsection 3: Authorities of Medical Society

In the contemporary medical world, whenever a novel treatment is discovered, it is publicized through world-famous journals, such as *Nature, Science, Lancet*, and more. Doctors and students get up-to-date knowledge from these journals.

I wrote an article demonstrating my discovery and submitted it to the above journals. Strangely, they gave me no reply as to whether they were going to accept my article for publication. If my article was imperfect, they ought to have notified me of the imperfection. They simply kept silent without stating a proper reason why they would not publish it.

Why did they do so? I cannot help thinking that it is due to the circumstance of the global medical community, as mentioned earlier. My method is too simple, too clear-cut, and yet completely effective for the world to behave normally. If it were more complicated and harder to understand, the possibility of acceptance for publication of the article should have been higher.

Let's explain with an easy example. Suppose a group of experts were studying how to make a room brighter. An expert would say, "Room arrangement is not good." Another one may say, "Wall color may be responsible." Still another one may suggest to change floor panels to a reflective one. Then a nonexpert joins the group and says, "More bulbs will make the room brighter." The problem may be solved by the nonexpert's idea, but experts won't be pleased because it makes them lose their status.

In the contemporary medical world, highly sophisticated theories are pursued, and basic and rudimentary points are overlooked. There is a proverb, "Lookers-on see most of the game." Sometimes persons seriously considering the problems don't realize the solution, but relaxed onlookers can solve it.

Although I have participated in medical research and clinical medicine for fifty years, you may say that I am a nonexpert in the field of immunology. From the viewpoint of global authorities in this field, their admission of nonexperts' discovery would deprive all experts of their positions and also bring about the loss of their research focus. Accordingly, they intend to prevent the publication of my article by all means. They must be hoping that things will go on as if nothing has changed.

Under these circumstances, I gave up publishing an article in the medical world for a while and decided to publish it in the pharmacological world. Consequently, my article has been published in *Pharmacometrics*, whose editorial office is located in the campus of the Tohoku University. The article is shown in subsection nine of this chapter. *Pharmacometrics* is an authoritative journal in the field of pharmacy.

In the end, my idea seems to be admitted in the pharmacological world but not in the medical world. As far as I am concerned, I have no intention of self-propagandizing, and it does not matter at all whether my idea is admitted, but it is most regrettable that no other doctors know about this treatment.

All physicians in the world would come to know about it if it is published in a world-famous journal in the field of medicine. Then the patients not only in Japan but also throughout the whole world could be saved. Nothing is as regrettable as this. However, a negative pessimism improves nothing. I decided to inform you directly through this book.

Subsection 4: Circumstances of This Discovery

Now I would like to explain how I came to find this method. For details, you may take a look at my article in subsection nine.

Have you ever heard of a story that parasite carriers seldom become allergic?

In 1988, a middle-aged man suffering from bronchial asthma came to my clinic. I chose an intracutaneous injection with Asthremedin (see the article), thinking that it would be more radical than other treatments. The injection was more effective than I had expected, but the mechanism of action of Asthremedin was unknown. The manufacturer of Asthremedin explained the mechanism, standing on an old, incorrect concept that unbalanced autonomic nerves caused the allergy. I kept this case in the back of my mind.

Three years later, NHK broadcasted a special program on pollen allergy. In the program, the hypothesis of Professor Sohmei Kojima, Department of Parasitology, University of Tokyo, Institute for Medical Sciences, was as follows: The reason why parasite carriers seldom suffer from allergic diseases may be because antiparasite antibodies occupy the receptors of antibodies on the surface of mast cells of the carriers. Simultaneously upon hearing the hypothesis, an idea flashed in my mind. In my previous case, the Asthremedin must have acted the role of parasites.

Thus I finally discovered how to cure not only allergic diseases but also allergic diathesis. However, how to cure collagen diseases remained unsolved. Fortunately, collagen diseases are caused by a similar mechanism as allergic diseases. Both diseases take place when pathogen-specific antibodies attach to responsible cells. The responsible cells are mast cells in cases of allergic diseases, and cytolytic T lymphocites (killer cells) in cases of collagen diseases.

It didn't take me much time to realize that both sorts of diseases can be cured by an identical method.

By the way, pathogen-specific antibodies are antibodies of allergens, which are substances causing allergic symptoms or physical stimuli, which in turn cause allergic symptoms, such as warmness, coldness, and ultra-violet rays in cases of allergic diseases. In cases of collagen diseases, they are antibodies of an organ of the patient; hence they are called autoantibodies.

Subsection 5: Outline of This Method

If I dared to name the method described above, I would call it antibody substitution method.

Generally, doctors keep in mind an old, incorrect concept that antibodies don't substitute for each other. The present discovery may be regarded as a controversial assertion in the contemporary world of medicine—a reason why my article won't be accepted by medical journals.

In the world of pharmacy, writers submit an article to *Pharmacometrics* before they apply to the Ministry of Health, Welfare, and Labor for admission of a drug. Therefore, no drug is admitted without an article published in this journal. To be admitted by the ministry, no less than 30 percent effect of a drug tested on animals is necessary.

As I stated above, my article was not accepted by medical journals, and I was obliged to submit it to *Pharmacometrics*, which published it. The article referee, who was a pharmacologist, recognized and appraised the relevancy of my idea.

My method is to accumulate nonspecific antibodies in the bodies of patients of allergic or collagen diseases. How this accumulation works is as follows: Mutual substitutions between accumulated new, normal, nonspecific antibodies and old, pathogen-specific antibodies take place to an extent depending on the quantity of the accumulation. When the accumulation reaches a sufficient level, all of the old pathogen-specific antibodies dissociate from the responsible cells, bringing about the extinction of the cause of the disease. Where there is no cause, there is no disease.

Practically, a necessary and sufficient condition for the accumulation of normal, nonspecific antibodies is to repeatedly inject the patient with normal, nonspecific antigens intradermally. The reason why the injection has to be intradermal is because the injected antigen has to stay in the subcutaneous tissue long enough to have the tissue produce antibodies.

Subsection 6: Pertinent Symptoms and Diseases

Concerning collagen diseases, which are regarded as incurable and of which satisfactory treatment has not been established, symptoms are so various that you cannot specify them as diseases with certain symptoms. Because the immune strength of the patient injures a part of the patient's body, an injured part or abnormal data of blood tests help you identify collagen diseases.

Recently, the number of people who have allergies is increasing due to aggravations of food and environment. Atopic dermatitis is an allergic disease, but from another point of view, there is an explanation that it is a collagen disease, in which the skin is injured. The treatment that is being carried out for collagen diseases today is to use immune-suppressing agents and/or steroid hormones. They may improve the symptom temporarily but are not actual cures.

Rheumatoid arthritis has existed for a long time, and it mainly appears among elderly women. Recently, the number of cases involving younger people has been increasing. The early symptoms are morning stiffness in the hands and fingers and pain in the knee, especially when descending stairways. There is no treatment that heals rheumatoid arthritis completely—except the one, of which I am informing you now.

Subsection 7: Completely Recovered Cases

Twenty years have passed since I found this method and started applying it to clinical practice. During this period, I have treated more than 550 cases of various allergic diseases, nearly 60 cases of autoimmune (collagen) diseases, and nearly 30 cases of a combination of the both diseases. The relevancy of this method has been proved by these results of my clinical practice.

In all cases, except for those who dropped out of the treatment, the diseases were completely cured after repeated intradermal injections with nonspecific antigens.

There are broad individual differences among my results. The case of perfect recovery after the least number of injections was a fifty-one-year-old woman, who recovered after only one injection. This is an unbelievable and extremely encouraging example. She had had morning stiffness in all fingers for two weeks, a typical symptom of rheumatoid arthritis. She came to my clinic once and received only one injection. I talked to her over the telephone twenty-one months later, and she said that she had been free of any symptom since the injection.

On the other end of the spectrum, the case of the lowest efficiency was an 18-month-old girl suffering from atopic dermatitis, who recovered after 194 injections given during 21 months. An explanation for this sort of difference would be that the girl had had atopic dermatitis since almost immediately after her birth; hence she was inherently allergic and should have had a large quantity of pathogen-specific antibodies. The rheumatoid woman received the injection at an early point of two weeks after the onset of her subjective symptom, and the quantity of pathogen-specific antibodies was small enough to be substituted by the normal, nonspecific antibodies produced after only one injection.

I would like to describe thirty typical cases in detail below.

Case 1. Sixty-nine-year-old female. First treated on September 18, 1991.

Patient spent seven weeks around the fumes of incense ten months ago. A month later, she caught a cold and did not get better for two months. Five months after that, she suffered from dyspnoea. A month thereafter, a doctor diagnosed her with emphysema. Another month later, she visited my clinic. Chest X-rays showed reticular shadows over all lung fields, right lung being worse than the left. I diagnosed her with interstitial pneumonia. She received intradermal injections with Asthremedin (see the article shown in subsection nine) at intervals of two to three days for nine months, increasing the injection dose gradually. The initial dose of injected protein was 1.4 mg, and the final dose was 18 mg. Her dyspnoea was better as of June 20, 1992.

Case 2. Twenty-five-year-old female. First treated on January 31, 1992.

Patient experienced urticaria after a high intake of shrimp in her childhood. For several years, she had alcoholic hepatitis and hepatitis B. She had an urticaria of unknown origin for three days. She received a total of 33 intradermal injections with Asthremedin during a period of 130 days. The initial dose was 1.4 mg, and the final was 6.6 mg. Afterward, she had no urticaria.

On November 29, 2002, her type IV collagen, 7S (a specific blood test for liver cirrhosis) showed 5.4 ng/ml (a normal person should not have more than 5.0). She received a total of 103 intradermal injections with Asthremedin during a period of 70 months. The initial dose was 3 μg, and the final dose was 26 mg.

Results of a follow-up of type IV collagen, 7S, were as follows: 5.0 ng/ml on October 14, 2003; 5.3 ng/ml on February 16, 2004; 5.5 ng/ml on April 13, 2004; 5.4 ng/ml on September 6, 2004; 5.1 ng/ml on March 7, 2005; 5.0 ng/ml on June 27, 2005; 4.8 ng/ml on August 19, 2005; 4.0 ng/ml on March 27, 2006; 4.7 ng/ml on October 26, 2006; 4.4 ng/ml on January 25, 2007; and 4.0 ng/ml on August 11, 2008.

Case 3. Forty-six-year-old female. First treated on January 7, 1993.

Patient was diagnosed with hyperthyroidism at her employer's medical examination twenty-eight years ago. She had been taking Thyamazol for all of those years. She had urticaria when she was mentally anxious, as well as muscle cramps in the chest or in the calf, and she was easily fatigued.

She received a total of 337 intradermal injections with Asthremedin from the start date listed above through October 27, 2004. The initial dose was 1.4 mg and the final was 4.4 mg. On June 16, 2008, I confirmed absence of recurrence.

Case 4. Fifty-five-year-old female. First treated on November 16, 1993.

Patient had nocturnal and morning stiffness and edema of the fingers for three months. Under the diagnosis of rheumatoid arthritis, she received a total of four intradermal injections with Asthremedin of 1.4 mg at intervals of one to two days. On June 16, 2008, I confirmed absence of recurrence.

Case 5. Sixty-four-year-old female. First treated on January 25, 1994.

Patient had discolored (dark gray) nails for approximately ten years. Her blood antinuclear antibody was 320x on December 1, 1997 (normally it is less than 40x). She had itchiness around her waist when she was in a hot bath. Under diagnosis of collagen disease of the nail and heat-allergic dermatitis, she had been receiving intradermal injections with Neurotropin, a product of Nippon Zohki Pharmaceutical Company consisting of extract of rabbit skin infected and inflamed with Vaccinia virus, at intervals of three to four days for over sixteen years. Her nail color and the itchiness healed. Her antinuclear antibody value improved to nearly normal range temporarily from November, 2006 to February, 2008. However, it resumed the abnormally high value (320x) thereafter presumably because I reduced the injection dosage, obeying the demand of the patient, who did not like vigorous skin reactions to the injection.

Case 6. Fifty-one-year-old female. First treated on September 12, 1991.

Patient had morning stiffness in all fingers, as well as edema and difficulty in bending the right hand fingers for two weeks. Under the diagnosis of rheumatoid arthritis, she received an intradermal injection with Asthremedin of 1.4 mg. She was free from any subjective symptom as of June 8, 1993.

Case 7. Fifty-eight-year-old male. First treated on November 10, 1993.

Patient used to have urticaria after drinking alcohol in his youth. He had morning stiffness in all fingers for a year. Under diagnosis of allergic diathesis and rheumatoid arthritis, he received an intradermal injection with Asthremedin of 1.4 mg protein. On June 16, 2008, I confirmed absence of recurrence.

Case 8. Forty-year-old male. First treated on September 14, 1994.

The patient had ongoing condition in childhood. After growing up, he had approximately one attack of bronchial asthma yearly, daily morning stiffness of all fingers, and intermittent edema of all fingers and both knees. Under diagnosis of bronchial asthma and rheumatoid arthritis, he received a total of three intradermal injections with Asthremedin of 1.4 mg at intervals of four to five days. On June 16, 2008, I confirmed absence of recurrence.

Case 9. Forty-eight-year-old male. First treated on March 9, 1995.

Patient had eye itchiness, tears, sneezing, and coryza in early spring for a couple of years. Under diagnosis of cedar-pollen allergy, he received a total of forty intradermal injections with Asthremedin (initially 1.4 mg and finally 19.8 mg) until June 27, 1995. He was free from any symptoms until April 1996, when he had pain in both elbows and the third joint of the fourth finger of the right hand. Under diagnosis of rheumatoid arthritis, he received a total of twenty-five intradermal injections with Asthremedin (initially 1.4 mg and finally 4.4 mg) until December 28, 1996. The pain disappeared.

Case 10. Fifty-five-year-old female. First treated on October 23, 1995.

Patient claimed pain in the third joint of her left small finger and the second joint of her right small finger that had gradually worsened for the last ten years. She also had sneezing and coryza upon going outside for the last five years. She received an intradermal injection with one ampoule of Kohtamin (see the article published from *Pharmacometrics*) under the diagnosis of rheumatoid arthritis and cold-allergic rhinitis. On June 16, 2008, I confirmed absence of recurrence.

Case 11. Sixty-two-year-old male. First treated on November 8, 1996.

Patient claimed a cold feeling of his right calf when going to sleep and a swelling of his right knee for over ten years, difficulty bending his right knee for six months, and reddish spots on both arms and legs that become itchy upon scratching for eight months. Under the diagnosis of rheumatoid arthritis and atopic dermatitis, he received a total of thirteen intradermal injections with Kohtamin with or without Asthremedin (initial dose 3 μg of Kohtamin and final dose 10 μg of Kohtamin plus 0.4 mg of Asthremedin) during a period of forty-eight days. At the time of the last injection, he informed me of improvement of his subjective symptoms.

Case 12. Forty-seven-year-old male. First treated on May 31, 1997.

In May 1995, patient underwent a medical examination and was diagnosed with hyperthyroidism, idiopathic thrombocytopenia, and autoimmune hepatitis. He received treatment with steroid hormones but did not heal completely. In my clinic, he received a total of one hundred intradermal injections with Asthremedin (initial dose 75 μg and final dose 13 mg) until October 6, 1998. Thereafter, he voluntarily stopped receiving the treatment until November 21, 1999. On November 22, 1999, he came to my clinic and said that his urinary protein was very strongly positive at his yearly checkup. Under diagnosis of nephrotic syndrome, he received a total of sixty-seven intradermal injections with Asthremedin (initial dose 3 μg and final dose 4.4 mg) during the period from November 22, 1999, to September 13, 2001. Thereafter, he again voluntarily stopped receiving treatment until October 11, 2002, when he came to my clinic. The test of his urinary protein revealed strongly positive. He resumed receiving intradermal injections with Asthremedin four times until October 22, 2002 (initial dose 3 μg and final dose 7 μg). He once again voluntarily stopped receiving treatment until June 9, 2005, when he resumed the treatment. He received a total of fifty-one intradermal injections with Kohtamin until March 15, 2006 (initial dose 0.01 μg and final dose 0.045 μg). The blood test on March 15, 2006, revealed complete recoveries of all of his diseases except for nephrotic syndrome. He had no subjective symptoms.

Case 13. Sixty-seven-year-old female. First treated on September 27, 1996.

Patient claimed pain in both knees for two months and pain in both foot joints for one month. Under the diagnosis of rheumatoid arthritis, she received a total of twenty-two intradermal injections with Kohtamin during a period of ten weeks (initial dose 2 μg and final dose 12 μg). Thereafter, a total of forty-two intradermal injections with Asthremedin were given during a period of twenty-four weeks (initial dose 1.4 mg and final dose 3.6 mg). On June 16, 2008, I confirmed absence of recurrence.

Case 14. Forty-four-year-old female. First treated on June 15, 1998.

Patient claimed a cold feeling even in the summer for the last three years. Her normal temperature was below thirty-six degrees centigrade; it was likely that she had a low basal metabolic rate. I was suspicious of hypothyroidism and checked her thyroid function. Her TSH (thyroid stimulating hormone) was within normal limit, and both of the thyroid hormones were close to the lower normal limit. Under diagnosis of hypopituitary hypothyroidism, she received a total of one hundred thirty intradermal injections with Asthremedin during seventeen months (initial dose 15 μg and final dose 13 mg). On October 1, 2009, I confirmed absence of recurrence.

Case 15. Sixty-two-year-old female. First treated on October 31, 1998.

Patient claimed allergic symptoms against pollens of cedar, Japanese cypress, and more for seven years, as well as edema on both knees and both foot joints for seven months. Five months before visiting me, she had been admitted to the orthopedics department of a hospital and was treated with steroid hormones. Her edema improved, leaving liquid accumulations in the joint spaces. Under diagnosis of pollen allergy and rheumatoid arthritis, I gave her a total of 215 intradermal injections with Asthremedin during the next nineteen months (initial dose 3 μg and final dose 9 mg). She was free from any sign of recurrence as of June 16, 2008.

Case 16. Thirty-one-year-old female. First treated on November 4, 1998.

In 1987, the patient had an abnormally high level of blood rheumatoid factor but ignored it. Eight years later, she had morning stiffness of her right forefinger, was diagnosed with rheumatoid arthritis, and was given Loxoprofen Sodium; her symptoms worsened. Two months later, another physician gave her Bucillamine, Diclofenac Sodium, and Etodolac. These medicines caused eczema, vomiting, headache, fever, pain in both arms and both legs, and difficulty walking. She immediately visited a third physician, who gave her a Chinese medicine and subcutaneously injected her with sodium thiomalate gold for three years.

In my clinic, she received a total of sixty-four intracutaneous injections with Asthremedin at intervals of two to five days during the period from November 4, 1998, to May 15, 1999 (initial dose 3 μg and final dose 29 mg). As of June 16, 2008, she rarely had dull pain in her fingers and toes and did not have any inconvenience in her daily life.

Case 17. Eighty-nine-year-old female. First treated on June 23, 1999.

Patient claimed morning stiffness of all fingers and pain in her left knee for three weeks. Under diagnosis of rheumatoid arthritis, she received a total of forty-nine intracutaneous injections with Asthremedin during a period of four months and one week (initial dose 3 μg protein and final dose 2.2 mg). She was free of any sign of recurrence as of June 16, 2008.

Case 18. Fifty-five-year-old female. First treated on July 2, 1999.

Patient claimed easy fatigability and dull headache for over ten years. Her tongue was thick and wide. She had had a husky voice for a long time. She sometimes was unable to speak. Suspecting hypothyroidism, I checked her thyroid function. Both her TSH and thyroid hormones were within normal limit, but all of them were close to the lower limits; the diagnosis was hypopituitary hypothyroidism. Under the diagnosis, she received a total of five intracutaneous injections with Asthremedin during the period from July 9, 1999 to July 19, 1999 (initial dose 3 μg and final dose 15 μg). She was free of any sign of recurrence as of June 16, 2008.

Case 19. Fifty-one-year-old female. First treated on September 17, 1999.

Patient claimed morning stiffness of all fingers for six months. Under diagnosis of rheumatoid arthritis, she received a total of nineteen intradermal injections with Asthremedin during the period from September 17, 1999 to November 20, 1999 (initial dose 3 μg and final dose 1.1 mg). She was free from any sign of recurrence as of June 16, 2008.

Case 20. Seventy-seven-year-old female. First treated on February 28, 2000.

Patient claimed that she had had wheezing coughs before her night sleep for three weeks. She had no other symptoms. Under diagnosis of bronchial asthma, she received a total of twenty-six intradermal injections with Asthremedin during the next three months (initial dose 3 μg and final dose 4.4 mg). Thereafter, she voluntarily stopped receiving treatment until October 2, 2000, when she resumed the treatment claiming that she had had morning stiffness of all fingers for six weeks and that she had had pain in her right knee for several days. Under diagnosis of complication of rheumatoid arthritis, she received a total of fifty-three intradermal injections with Asthremedin during the next five months and three weeks (initial dose 1.4 mg and final dose 8.8 mg). She was free from any subjective symptoms as of June 16, 2008.

Case 21. Sixty-six-year-old male. First treated on April 8, 2000.

Patient was diagnosed with nephrotic syndrome on March 11, 2000. He received a total of twenty-six intradermal injections with Asthremedin during the next three months and nine days (initial dose 3 μg and final dose 2.2 mg). He was free from any subjective symptoms as of June 16, 2008.

Case 22. Twenty-five-year-old female. First treated on July 2, 2004.

Patient claimed an edema in her left mandibular area for three days. Her blood test revealed that her TSH was within normal range and that the levels of her thyroid hormones were abnormally low; she had hypopituitary hypothyroidism. She received a total of eleven intradermal injections with 0.1 ml of Neurotropin during the next twenty-four days. She was free from any symptoms as of June 16, 2008.

Case 23. Forty-one-year-old female. First treated on December 13, 2004.

Patient had had morning stiffness and pain of all fingers seven years ago. She had morning stiffness, pain, and edema of all fingers for the last six weeks. Under diagnosis of rheumatoid arthritis, she received a total of twenty-three intradermal injections with 0.1 ml of Neurotropin during the next two months and nine days. She was free from any symptom as of June 16, 2008.

Case 24. Forty-nine-year-old female. First treated on May 9, 2005.

Patient had morning stiffness of both thumbs for one month and a persistent cough for a couple of days. Under diagnosis of rheumatoid arthritis and bronchial asthma, she received a total of nineteen intradermal injections with Neurotropin during the next five months and ten days (initially 0.1 ml and finally 0.2 ml). She was free from any symptoms as of June 16, 2008.

Case 25. Seventy-eight-year-old female. First treated on February 25, 2006.

Patient had morning stiffness of all fingers for a year and pain in both knees for six months. Under diagnosis of rheumatoid arthritis, she received an intradermal injection with 0.1 ml of Neurotropin on the day of her first treatment. She was free of any symptoms as of June 16, 2008.

Case 26. Seventy-year-old female. First treated on June 23, 2006.

Patient had morning and evening stiffness of all fingers, with evenings being worse than mornings and her right hand fingers being worse than the left, for ten years. She also had pain in the left knee for a week. Under diagnosis of rheumatoid arthritis, she received a total of fifty-one intradermal injections with Neurotropin during the next five months (initially 0.1 ml and finally 0.6 ml). She was free from any symptoms as of June 16, 2008.

Case 27. Fifty-eight-year-old female. First treated on March 29, 2007.

Patient had easy fatigability for several months. Her tongue was thick, and her normal temperature was 34.6 degrees centigrade, indicating a low basal metabolic rate and hypothyroidism. Her TSH was abnormally high, and both thyroid hormones were abnormally low. Under diagnosis of hypothyroidism, she received a total of eleven intradermal injections with Neurotropin during the next four weeks (initially 0.1 ml and finally 0.14 ml). She was free of any symptoms as of June 16, 2008.

Case 28. Sixty-eight-year-old female. First treated on November 9, 2007.

Patient claimed that she was extraordinarily sensitive to cold environments and had poor memory. Her mother and younger sister had hypothyroidism. Results of her thyroid function test indicated her TSH was abnormally high, and both thyroid hormones were within normal limits but close to the lower limits. Under diagnosis of hypothyroidism, she received a total of seventeen intradermal injections with 0.1 ml of Neurotropin during the next thirty-eight days. She was free from any symptoms as of June 16, 2008.

Case 29. Fifty-three-year-old female. First treated on October 28, 2008.

Patient had pain in her right knee that became severe upon descending stairways for three weeks. Under diagnosis of rheumatoid arthritis, she received a total of fifty-six intradermal injections with

Neurotropin during the next four months and nineteen days. The injection dose was raised by 40 percent every eleventh time (initially 0.1 ml and finally 0.56 ml). She was free from any symptoms as of October 1, 2009.

Case 30. Fifty-year-old female. First treated on October 18, 2008.

Patient claimed that she had been easily fatigued for four months and that she had edema in both sides of mandibular areas since that morning. Her tongue was thick, and the inside of her mouth, including the throat, looked edematous as a whole. Her pulse rate was 58 and her normal temperature was 35.4 degrees centigrade, indicating a low basal metabolic rate. Results of her thyroid function test were within normal limits, but the thyroid hormones were close to the lower limits. Under diagnosis of hypopituitary hypothyroidism, she received a total of twenty-one intradermal injections with Neurotropin during the next seven weeks (initially 0.1 ml and finally 0.2 ml). She was free of any symptoms during the last week of treatment.

Although I have described thirty cases above, I still have a number of similar cases in which collagen diseases, with or without complications of allergic diseases, healed completely. The number of injections varied according to the severity of the disease. The more severe the disease, the higher number of injections required. It is important to be persistent.

In addition, this method gives no side effects because it uses harmless antigens only.

Subsection 8: Possible Applications of This Method

I would now like to address the possible application of the antibody substitution method.

Rejection of organ transplants could be prevented by a large quantity of nonspecific antibodies that have been accumulated in the body of the recipient before the transplantation. The speculated mechanism of the prevention is as follows: The antibody receptors on the surface of killer cells will be saturated by nonspecific antibodies after their accumulation. After the transplantation, antibodies against the organ will be produced in the recipient, but their quantity will be smaller than those of nonspecific antibodies. Therefore few, if any, antibodies against the organ will attach to killer cells. Consequently, little, if any, rejection will take place.

Amyotrophic lateral sclerosis (ALS) could also be cured by this method. However, no practical proof has yet been obtained for either situation.

Subsection 9: The Article Published in *Pharmacometrics*

応用薬理 Oyō Yakuri

Pharmacometrics 76(5/6) 105-107 (2009)   105

Therapeutic Significance of Non-Specific Antigens As
Anti-Allergic and Anti-Autoimmune Agents

Kimihiko Okazaki[*]

Okazaki Medical Clinic, 62 Azekatsucho, Nishikyogoku, Ukyoku, Kyoto 615-0806, Japan

Received April 27, 2009. Accepted June 29, 2009

The usefulness of non-specific antigens in treatments of immune diseases is demonstrated. The results of clinical practices applying the above concept on 645 cases *in toto* were almost perfect, the only exception being those who dropped out of the treatment.

Keywords: Antigen/Antibody/Specificity/Substitution

Introduction

No one can deny that contemporary Medicine has made remarkable progress. However, some diseases such as cancers, autoimmune diseases, acquired immunodeficiency syndrome(AIDS), and even allergic diseases remain hard to cure completely. Fortunately, the author was able to find an extremely simple theory that might solve a part of the above problems, i.e. how to cure allergic and autoimmune diseases completely. This theory is based on a unique viewpoint, details of which follow.

It is well established that injected antigens give rise to antibodies that are complementary to the antigens. It is also well established that an equilibrium state exists between antibodies that are in the vicinity of their receptors on the cell-surfaces. That is that some antibodies are attached to the receptors and some others are not although there are ceaseless position-changes. In other words, every antibody molecule continuously attaches, detaches, and re-attaches to its receptors. The reason why it is not "its receptor" but "its receptors" is because every antibody molecule may change receptors. On the other hand, it is well known that allergic diseases are caused by combinations of mast cells and allergen-specific antibodies. It is also well known that autoimmune diseases are caused by combinations of cytolytic T-lymphocytes and organ-

[*]Correspondence author: Kimihiko Okazaki, M.D., Ph.D
Okazaki Medical Clinic, 62 Azekatsucho, Nishikyogoku, Ukyoku, Kyoto 615-0806
Tel: +81-75-314-8123; Fax: +81-75-314-8123
E-mail: ons13082.x@kmail.nsilkyou.ne.jp

specific antibodies.

The question is whether these combinations, or partnerships, could be broken off because it is obvious that the diseases would be cured if they could. Fortunately, the author happened to discover the answer to the above question, which is, "Yes" in fact. The clue to the discovery was the so-called Kojima theory (Sohuzi Kojima, 1979), i.e. "The reason why parasite-carriers seldom suffer from allergic diseases may be because anti-parasite antibodies saturate the antibody-receptors on the surface of parasite-carriers' mast cells." This theory was presented as an explanation of the experience of Turton (J.A. Turton, 1976), who had cured his own chronic pollen allergy by a 3-time repetition of infections and exterminations of hookworms. What I thought upon hearing about these circumstances was that Turton must have had anti-pollen antibodies before he has obtained anti-hookworm antibodies because he had had a pollen allergy for 30 years when he first infected himself with hookworm. Another important point is that the 3-time repetition was necessary for him to cure the allergy. That means that the quantity of anti-hookworm antibodies must have been large enough to compete with his anti-pollen antibodies for their receptors and to defeat them in order to take over the position of anti-pollen antibodies on their receptors on the surface of his mast cells. In other words, there must have been mutual substitutions of antibodies on the receptors on the surface of mast cells. In accord with this concept are the following articles: Stanworth *et al.*

27

1967, Ishizaka *et al.* 1973, Bazaral *et al.* 1973, Godfrey, 1975, Knapp *et al.* 1985, Hässig, 1986, De Simone *et al.* 1988, Rakestraw *et al.* 1992, and Nydegger *et al.* 2000. This mechanism of antibodies' mutual substitutions could be applied to treatments of autoimmune diseases as well as to those of allergic diseases, both of which have a similar etiology, i.e. specific antibodies cooperate with cytolytic T lymphocytes in autoimmune diseases while they cooperate with mast cells in allergic diseases.

Methods

To apply the above concept to treatments of allergic and autoimmune diseases, it would only be necessary to accumulate non-specific antibodies in the patients' bodies. In order to do so, repetition of intracutaneous injections with non-specific antigens would be necessary and sufficient. In order to avoid the severe pain of intracutaneous injection, 1/5 volume of 1% lidocaine solution was mixed with the non-specific antigen preparation.

Results and Discussion

Relevancy of the above concept has been proved by results of clinical practices during the last 18 years on 558 cases of various allergic diseases, 59 cases of various autoimmune diseases, and 28 cases of combinations of both types of the diseases, 645 *in toto*, all of which were completely cured after repetitions of intracutaneous injections with non-specific antigen preparations, except for those who dropped out of the treatment. Every treatment was given after an informed consent. Table 1 shows summary of 558 cases of allergic diseases and Tables 2 and 3 show those of 59 and 28 cases of autoimmune diseases without and with complication of allergic diseases, respectively. The numbers in the parentheses in Tables 1, 2, and 3 indicate percentages of recoveries calculated assuming that cases of "Unverifiable" and "Deceased of other cause" were absent. Apparently, it is safe to say that cases of "Almost perfect recovery" would have been "Literally perfect recovery" if the patients had not stopped receiving treatment voluntarily.

The details of a representative case are as follows: A 62-year-old woman claimed on April 2, 1999 that she had had a cedar pollen allergy for 3 years and that she had had a morning stiffness of all fingers, edema of both feet, and intermittent pain in the both hand joints for 3 months. Her rheumatoid factor on the same day was 93U/ml, the normal range being not more than 35U/ml. Diagnosis was cedar pollen allergy and rheumatoid arthritis. She received a total of 28 intracutaneous injections with Asthremedin, a product of Nippon Zohki Pharmaceutical Company, Osaka, consisting of extracts of rabbit's skin and testis, killed small pox viruses, fungi, and peptone with total protein of /ampoule(0.5ml) for series 1 and 2.2mg/ampoule(0.5ml) for series 2, in which the concentrations of all extracts except peptone were 3 times as high as those in the series 1. The initial dose was 3μg protein of Asthremedin, series 1. The site of injection was between the shoulder and elbow. The dose was raised by 50% every time until it reached 4.4mg protein; 2 ampoules of Asthremedin, series 2. Injection intervals were 2-6 days. She received the 27th injection on June 14, 1999 and was free from any subjective symptom until September 17, 1999 when she had pain in the soles of her feet. She received the 28th and the last injection with 2 ampoules of Asthremedin, series 2 on the same day. She notified me of her symptom-free state on June 15, 2000.

Table 1. Summary of 558 cases of allergic diseases

Extent of recovery	Cases	%		
Literally perfect recovery	243	43.6	58.1	(86.2)
Almost perfect recovery	81	14.5		
Dropped out of treatment	52	9.3		
Deceased of other cause	8	1.4		
Unverifiable	174	31.2		

Table 2. Summary of 59 cases of autoimmune diseases without complication of allergic diseases

Extent of recovery	Cases	%		
Literally perfect recovery	25	42.4	56.0	(66.0)
Almost perfect recovery	8	13.6		
Dropped out of treatment	17	28.8		
Deceased of other cause	1	1.6		
Unverifiable	8	13.6		

Table 3. Summary of 28 cases of autoimmune diseases with complication of allergic diseases

Extent of recovery	Cases	%		
Literally perfect recovery	11	39.3	60.7	(77.2)
Almost perfect recovery	6	21.4		
Dropped out of treatment	5	17.9		
Unverifiable	6	21.4		

Another representative case is a 20-month-old girl suffering from atopic dermatitis since almost immediately after the birth. She started receiving intracutaneous injections on June 5, 2007 with 0.01pg protein of Kohtamin, a product of Iboyu Pharmaceutical Company, Osaka, consisting of 20μg protein per ampoule(1ml) of killed *Neisseria sicca et flava*. Injection intervals were 2-3 days. The injection dose was raised by 40% every 20 times because her dermatitis worsened when the dose was raised at the 11th injection. The reason why the initial dose had to be as small as 0.01pg protein and why 20-time repetition of the same dose was necessary must be because atopic infants are much less capable of producing antibodies than non-atopic grown-ups. She received the 146th injection on July 22, 2008 when her skin condition was almost normal.

Some are of the opinion that intravenous infusion of non-specific γ-globulin should be much more effective than intracutaneous injections with non-specific antigens. However, infusion of γ-globulin has a definitive drawback, i.e. infused globulin is "non-self," consequently, anti-globulin antibodies would be produced in the recipient's body, which may cause an anaphylactic reaction after a number of infusions. On the contrary, non-specific antibodies that are produced after intracutaneous injections with antigens are "self," therefore, no anti-antibody antibodies would be produced however many times the injection may be repeated.

Acknowledgement

The author is grateful to Lecturer Michael E. Iunentz, Kyoto University Faculty of Literature, for his advice and reviewing the manuscript.

References

Bazaral, M., Orgel, H.A., and Hamburger, R.N. (1973): The influence of serum IgE levels of selected recipients, including patients with allergy, Helminthiasis and tuberculosis, on the apparent P-K titre of a reaginic serum. *Clin. Exp. Immunol.* 14, 117-125.

De Simone, C., Delogu, G., Corbetta,G.(1988):Intravenous immunoglobulins in association with antibiotics: a therapeutic trial in specific intensive care unit patients. *Crit. Care Med.* Jan; 16(1), 23-6.

Godfrey, R.C. (1975): Asthma and IgE levels in rural and urban communities in The Gambia. *Clinical Allergy*, 5, 201-207.

Hissig, A. (1986): Intravenous immunoglobulins: pharmacological aspects and therapeutic use. *Vox Sang.* 51(1), 10-7.

Ishizaka, T., Soto, C.S., and Ishizaka, K. (1973): Mechanisms of passive sensitization III. Number of IgE molecules and their receptor sites on human basophil granulocytes. *J. Immunol.* 111, 500-11.

Knapp, W., Majdic, O., Holter, W., Stockinger, H., and Köller, U. (1985): Considerations on the therapeutic use of monoclonal antibodies. *Wien Klin. Wochenschr.* 97(3), 97-107.

Kojima, S. (1979): Parasite diseases, IgE, and IgE antibodies, *Rinsho-I*, 5, 679.

Nydegger, U.E., Mohacsi, P.J., Escher, R., and Morell, A. (2000): Clinical use of intravenous immunoglobulins. *Vox Sang.* 78 Suppl 2, 191-5.

Ogawa, M., McIntyre, O.R., Ishizaka, K., Ishizaka, T., Terry, W.D., and Waldmann, T.A. (1971): Biologic properties of E myeloma proteins. *Amer. J. Med.* 51, 193-9.

Rakestraw, S.L., Ford, W.E., Tompkins, R.G., Rodgers, M.A., Thorpe, W.P., and Yarmush, M.L. (1992): Antibody-targeted photolysis: in vitro immunological, photophysical, and cytotoxic properties of monoclonal antibody-dextran-Sn(IV) chlorin e6 immunoconjugates. *Biotechnol. Prog.* 8(1), 30-9.

Stanworth, D.R., Humphrey, J.H., Bennich, H., and Johansson, S.G.O. (1967): Specific inhibition of the Prausnitz-Kuestner reaction by an atypical human melanoma protein. *Lancet*, ii, 330-2.

Turton, J.A. (1976): IgE, parasites, and allergy, *Lancet*, 2, 686.

CHAPTER 2:
Anti-cancer Agent with No Side Effects

You may remember that I said in the introduction of this book, "Why has an epoch-making treatment for cancer not been discovered when the number of cancer patients has grown so large?" But as a matter of fact, such a discovery was made and reported by a Japanese scholar, Dr. Mutsuyuki Kochi, as early as 1980. The clue of his discovery was, as he told me directly, obtained from the Old Testament. In more detail, a king of Israel developed a skin tumor, presumably melanoma, and his priest prayed for the king's recovery. The priest received a divine message that the king's tumor shall be healed by sticking dried figs on it. Dr. Kochi extracted a large amount of figs, collected the fraction of the extract that was adsorbed by active charcoal (testing for antitumor activity by means of Ehrlich's ascites hepatoma cells), and identified the effective factor as benzaldehyde. Because benzaldehyde is a volatile organic solvent, he had to change it into a water-soluble substance. In order to do so, he had a pharmaceutical industry prepare a few chemical compounds—that is, cyclodextrin benzaldehyde inclusion compound, benzylidene glucose, and sodium ascorbate benzaldehyde. He carried out a couple of clinical studies on the anticancer activity of the former two compounds and reported the results through "Cancer Treatment Reports," which was the bulletin of The National Cancer Institute in New York.

You may wonder why such a discovery has not spread itself throughout the world. A reason could be that Dr. Kochi tested the efficacy of the medicines with terminal cancer patients, and the results were not too dramatic—the overall objective response rate was 55 percent in the last report, which was published from the bulletin in 1985. In my opinion, a 55 percent response out of *terminal* cancer patients is superb. My opinion is that because Dr. Kochi was not a member of the group of cancer researchers, his work was nothing but a nuisance to the group members. In addition, an inexpensive material like benzaldehyde or its derivatives would not be a source of capital gain for the industries concerned.

An invaluable piece of information is that benzaldehyde itself is contained in raw almond according to *The Merck Index*. That means that eating several raw almonds daily could heal an early stage of cancer and could also be useful to prevent cancers. Larger quantities of almond ingestion could be effective for middle stages of cancers.

Another invaluable information that I can provide you with is that *p*-hydroxybenzaldehyde is a potent anticancer agent. It is water soluble, 1 g dissolving in 200 ml of water, but it has a disagreeable taste. Mixing with starch can make it much more bearable. The only caution you need to take is to take only a small dose because otherwise the blood vessels in the tumor might be ruptured together with the tumor tissue. After taking the small dose—which is 2.5 mg or less according to the severity of the disease; the more severe the disease, the less the dose—daily for three weeks, you should raise the dose by 40 percent. You should keep raising the dose by 40 percent after you have taken a same dose for three weeks. In my experience, the maximum dose was 15 g daily in the case of an early stage of lung cancer, and the patient recovered completely without any other treatments.

As for the mechanism of action of benzaldehyde and its derivatives, it is likely that they act as inhibitors of the enzyme tyrosine kinase, which is the key enzyme in the pathway of cancer development. The reason why they inhibit the enzyme is because several groups in the chemical structures of both compounds, tyrosine and benzaldehyde, are the same. The common groups are the benzene nucleus and the carbonyl group. *p*-Hydroxybenzaldehyde has another common group, the hydroxyl group, which is also present in tyrosine. That *p*-hydroxybenzaldehyde has three common groups with tyrosine, the substrate of enzyme tyrosine kinase, may be the reason why the medicine is such a potent anticancer agent. The reason why a compound of an analogous structure of the substrate inhibits the enzyme activity is because the substrate site of the enzyme misrecognizes and accepts the compound as the substrate so that the original substrate cannot attach to the substrate site.

Still additional invaluable information that I can provide you with is that Benfothiamine; a compound in which benzoyl group combines with thiamine (vitamin B_1), has an antitumor activity. Benzoyl group consists of benzene nucleus and carbonyl group(-CO), while benzaldehyde consists of benzene nucleus and aldehyde group(-CHO). Namely, a hydrogen atom is absent in –CO, while it is present in –CHO. As far as antitumor activity is concerned, the single hydrogen atom is not significant. Ten tablets of Benfothiamine, 25 mg per tablet, taken every ten days will successfully prevent cancer developments. In order to treat developed cancers, you'd better take only one tablet daily for three weeks and raise the dose by 50 percent every three weeks until it reaches thirty tablets daily. Then, switch the medicine to *p*-hydroxybenzaldehyde, 200 mg daily. After having taken a same dose for 3 weeks, raise the dose by 40 percent.

An alternative choice would be to undergo a surgical extirpation and prevent the possible recurrence of cancer completely with Benfothiamine. In case there is no remaining tumor after the surgery, you can take a large dose of the medicine such as twenty tablets every ten days. But in case there is a possibility of a part of the tumor remaining after the surgery, you'd better follow the way of gradual raising of the dose of Benfothiamine as described above.

Some of you may think that such a discovery can't be relevant because authoritative oncologists have not approved it. However, you ought to be very cautious not to fall into their snare. In other words, a conspiracy of the oncologists is behind the cover-up of this information to keep the public ignorant of the fact that a cure for cancer has been found. The aim of the conspiracy is to protect the oncologists from loss of social and academic status. Contemporary oncologists work toward the discovery of specific medicines for cancer. An achievement of such a discovery has been reported by Dr. Kochi. If the oncologists evaluate the achievement properly, all of their current works would be rendered meaningless. They are abusing their authority to protect their reputations and finances. Originally, the purpose of medicine was to heal mankind's diseases. But now, mankind is being held victim to those oncologists. It is obvious that this conspiracy must not last forever. The sooner it terminates, the better.

In order to convince those who are skeptical about my story, I would like to add a few words as follows: I am acquainted with an authoritative oncologist, who is an ex-president of The Japanese National Cancer Institute in Tokyo. He is definitely aware of Kochi's achievement. I know that he knows the efficacy of benzaldehyde derivatives. Not only he, but also all of other authoritative oncologists could not recognize the relevancy of Kochi's achievement. You may wonder why. In short, an ignoble human desire is entangled.

If they should recognize the relevancy of the achievement, all of research problems of global oncologists would cease to exist. This is the reason why an epoch-making discovery must not take place.

Those workers work hard days and nights to find a specific medicine for cancer. For the sake of the workers, it is not desirable that such a medicine is discovered and spreads to the whole world so easily.

It is inconceivable for an ordinary person that they work aiming at a novel treatment for cancer hoping that no epoch-making discovery does not take place. It is a typical self-contradiction.

Human beings have strived for truth and have built the contemporary civilization spending so many years and months. No one can deny that the attitude is still valid, today.

However, the invisible mind that controls the contemporary world is not a noble one based on justice. Therefore, you can say, "The contemporary world is seriously ill."

Those who possess power try hard to obtain more money and/or concessions. For them, nothing is more important than maintaining their concessions and/or comfortable environments. Neither truth nor justice can parallel to them.

Unless you admit this cruel reality, your lives are not safely secured. Namely, your lives, that should be saved if properly treated, would be exposed to danger of being shortened.

Most of medical doctors who work under the name of medicine, which is supposed to save human lives, treat and prescribe for their patients according to their knowledge and experience. Most of medical doctors are ignorant of the ignoble reality. Most of cancer patients believe that they have no choice but to undergo surgery or to take harmful cancer drugs.

Owing to these conditions, related facilities and people are guaranteed to handsome incomes. Pharmaceutical industries enjoy copious capital gains selling cancer drugs.

It doesn't matter whether a cancer drug is effective because cancer patients will take them obeying their doctors regardless of the medicine's efficacy.

Lately, at last, the number of patients, who are skeptical about taking those cancer drugs, is increasing. Formerly, cancer drugs were gold mines for pharmaceutical companies. Annual domestic Japanese total fee of medical treatments exceeds thirty trillion yen. The fund of health insurance that keeps increasing every year will become bankrupt sooner or later.

Most of cancer patients, as a matter of fact, sign an oath obeying their doctors to receive harmful treatments while struggling with bills of health insurance and/or of the hospitals. This is the pathway that most of those who were sentenced to have a cancer would follow.

I hope that you have understood the reason why I, who have witnessed the miserable reality as mentioned above, cannot feel like passing away to the other world without leaving any information about harmless and side-effect-free cancer drugs.

There is absolutely nothing I gain if I publish a book like this. I have literally no desire for fame nor for honor. The only motivation of mine to leave this book to the contemporary world is that I just can't help doing so because my conscience doesn't allow me to stay still.

Now, I would like to demonstrate four representative cases of cancer that healed completely with the aid of benzaldehyde derivatives.

Case 1. A 77-year-old woman was diagnosed at a local hospital to have a malignant tumor (Grawitz's tumor) on the cranial edge of her left kidney on October 19, 1989. She was advised to undergo a surgical treatment; a renal extirpation, but she refused it and visited my clinic. I prescribed her 2 tablets daily of S-benzoylthiamine monophosphate (commercial name: Biotamine: product of Sankyo Company, Osaka, Japan) containing 11 mg of benzoyl group (5.5 mg *per* tablet) for 4 months. I raised the dose to 3 tablets daily on February 19, 1990 and she kept taking the medicine for 5 more months. By the end of that period, she was healthy enough to be able to enjoy a group bus tour. Her daughter lately told me that the patient had passed away due to senility in 2004 at age of 92.

Case 2. A 60-year-old man underwent a surgical extirpation of melanoma on the bending side of the left thigh on November 13, 1993. I prescribed him 1 g daily of sodium bonzoate in order to prevent a recurrence of melanoma on December 1, 1994. I kept raising the dose gradually until it reached 5 g daily and the patient kept taking it until January 31, 2000. By that time, the melanin pigments, which used to show themselves on the surface of the operation-scar, faded away completely. He has had no recurrence as of July 15, 2010.

Case 3. A 41-year-old man claimed on November 16, 2005 that he had had a pain in the right upper region of the chest for two weeks. An X-ray showed a round shadow of 8 mm diameter. Neuron specific enolase, the tumor marker specific for lung cancer, was estimated to be 18 ng/ml (normally not more than 10 ng/ml). Under diagnosis of early stage of lung cancer, I prescribed him 1 tablet daily of S-benzoylthiamine monophosphate (commercial name: Biotowa; product of Towa Pharmaceutical Company, Osaka, Japan, containg 5.5 mg of benzoyl group *per* tablet) on the same day. I gradually raised the dose to 30 tablets daily during the next 6 months lest the blood vessels in the tumor get ruptured and cause intra-organic hemorrhage. On may 24, 2006, I replaced 30 tablets daily of Biotowa with 70 mg of *p*-hydroxybenzaldehyde, 1 g of which being dissolved in 200 ml of water. I also gradually raised the dose, namely, a same dose was given for 3 weeks and 40-50% raise was carried out after every 3 weeks. The final dose was 15 g daily, which started on September 17, 2009. By the end of that month, his lung cancer was proved to have healed completely by a local hospital. During the last 12 months, the medicine was given as mixture with starch in the ratio of 4 to 1, 1 being the medicine. The value of neuron specific enolase dropped to the normal range in the 3rd month of treatment and stayed there thereafter. I confirmed absence of recurrence as of April 13, 2011.

Case 4. A 63-year-old man was diagnosed by an urologist with an early stage of prostate cancer on June 15, 2011. Three days later, I prescribed him 5 mg *per* day of *p*-hydroxybenzaldehyde. I raised the dose by 40% every 3 weeks. On September 2, 2011, the patient notified me of the result of clinical examination which had turned out to prove the disappearance of the tumor. I instructed him to keep taking the medicine every 10 days at the dose of 14 mg in order to prevent recurrence of the diseases.

As you may have noticed in the second case above, sodium benzoate is also a harmless and side-effect-free cancer drug. That is because the essential factor of the drug is benzoyl group, which is a combination of a benzene nucleus and a carbonyl group (-CO), and benzoic acid has a hydroxyl group (-OH) combining to the carbonyl carbon of benzoyl group. Sodium benzoate has a sodium atom (Na) instead of hydrogen atom of OH in benzoic acid. As far as antitumor activity is concerned, these OH and ONa are not significant.

CHAPTER 3:

How to Control Overnourished States without Restricting Food Intake

In advanced countries, the rate of deaths due to diseases caused by atherosclerotic changes to blood vessels is worse than any other rate of deaths not due to blood vessel problems. The atherosclerotic changes include heart attacks, brain strokes, and the like. Atherosclerosis of blood vessels is caused by overnourishment. Diabetes mellitus (DM) is also caused by overnourishment, and aggravates atherosclerosis. Needless to say, restricting food intake requires a strong willpower. However, there is a way by which you can reduce your weight without strong willpower—the egg diet. Eggs consist of high-molecular-weight molecules, that is, proteins and nucleic acids with small quantities of carbohydrate and lipid. The former molecules are digested in the alimentary canal into low-molecular-weight compounds, such as amino acids and mononucleotides. The low-molecular-weight compounds enter the liver through the portal vein, which connects the alimentary canal with the liver. In the liver, the compounds are converted into high-molecular-weight molecules, consuming synthetic energies. In order to supply the synthetic energy, blood lipid, blood sugar, subcutaneous fat, and lipids on the inside wall of blood vessels are decomposed. Thus, you can lose weight and improve the state of blood vessels and of DM. The small quantity of lipid in egg yolk can be rendered poorly absorbed from the alimentary canal by boiling eggs hard. The fewer the number, the less the effect. The most desirable number of hard-boiled eggs to eat daily is twenty. As for the cholesterol contained in egg yolk, the liver enzyme, which is capable of decomposing cholesterol, decomposes the excessive cholesterol.

Although hard-boiled eggs are not too tasty, you should not put mayonnaise or other oily stuff on them. A way to make eggs tasty and hard is to heat mixed raw eggs in the microwave after mixing them with soy sauce or a similar stuff. You could also heat mixed raw eggs in a pan without adding oil. A way to make hard-boiled eggs admirably tasty is to soak them in saturated and chilled cooking salt water over-night without peeling the shell.

Alternatives to the egg diet are an essential amino acids mixture and casein. Their action mechanism is the same as the egg diet except that nucleic acids are absent in casein and in essential amino acids mixture. Practically, twenty to thirty grams daily is sufficient.

Mechanism of action of the protein diet was proposed by a West German athletic physiologist, whose name is Miguel Dobronsky, in 1981 or earlier.

The only drawback of egg-diet is a high possibility of getting gout. The reason is because nucleic acids in egg yolk can be converted to uric acid, crystals of which are the cause of gout. However, you always feel a dull pain in your thumb or in the first toe at the early stage of gout. Therefore, if you take a tablet or two of Benzmarone; an accelerator of excretion of uric acid, the dull pain should disappear and the early stage of gout should heal completely.

Assuming that you have regained your health, I will have more information that I wish to provide you with about how to prevent another illness. If you should get ill again, the information in the next chapter will tell you how to overcome it. It also will tell you how to maintain your physical health in a good condition.

Chapter 4:
Care of Mind

Subsection 1: Mind Rules Body

Human bodies do not just consist of physical bodies. The other constituent is the soul. Soul may remind you of religion, however, this is not a religious talk but a scientific truth.

Souls are invisible, and so today's science cannot identify them. A few people are able to see the appearance of soul as an aura. To those who declare, "Souls don't exist," I say they might as well state, "Minds don't exist." Naturally, minds are invisible to the eyes. X-rays cannot detect the mind, either. Can you still say that mind doesn't exist? If you had no mind, you would not be human.

Physical bodies have their own life spans; human beings must die sooner or later. People want to die without regrets and preferably without suffering from diseases. I would like you to understand the relationship between the physical body and the spirit as well as the relationship between the mind and the soul. We have been living too deeply attached to physical body. What supports your body is your soul; it is also the way how to control your mind.

What you should do in order to stay healthy is to keep your mind sound. It is important not to think pessimistically but to think positively. There is a statistic that lively people have a considerably lower probability of falling ill than melancholic people.

Some doctors say, "You'd better laugh if you don't want to die of cancer." Do not worry about the little things. I don't mean to be neglectful, but I mean to live in the way of "Que sera, sera." Everything goes on as it does. Nothing takes a favorable turn if you mope over trifles—rather, things may take an *unfavorable* turn if you mope over trifles. By consuming energy worrying about this and that, you end up with a worse result. Let's stop that practice now, because it doesn't pay at all.

As you know, there is a theory that normal cells are transformed into cancer cells by the actions of superactive oxygen. The alleged cause of the generation of superactive oxygen is stress. Unless you improve your way of living and stop receiving stresses, you will be prone to this kind of risk. It is not the body but the mind that feels stress.

Subsection 2: Wisdom for Survival in a Society Full of Stresses

Contemporary society is full of stresses. In big cities, people take crowded trains to arrive at their places of work before the fixed time. At home, there are often problems between the couple or between parent and child. None of the stress gets solved. In order to stay healthy, you ought to make yourself unsusceptible to stresses.

Among people, there are various ways of feeling about an incident. That is, some people don't interpret an ordinary stress as a stress. In order to be like them, you can choose the way "Que sera, sera." You won't necessarily get a good result even if you make more efforts than the average person. Just stop worrying and try to think, *I did my best. I leave the rest to heaven.*

If you find you can't switch yourself to this mentality, look for the reason why. Generally, human beings expect others to recognize what he or she has done. In addition, most people expect others to evaluate them more highly than their fellow workers. They want to be promoted earlier than fellow workers, with better wages; their families would then begin to respect them more, improving home circumstances.

This type of thinking centers on money. I previously wrote that in most, if not all, countries on this planet, people aspire to be rich. The reason why we are unable to live in the way of "Que sera, sera" is because we are too deeply attached to money.

Your stresses will not be dissolved as long as you keep thinking that the aim of life is to earn money in order to possess more money than others. Stresses from poverty also come from attachment to money. Although it's very difficult to live with absolutely no money, those who think, *Things will turn out one way or the other.* don't feel stressed even if they have very little money.

Those who have lived believing that money is more precious than their own lives ought to realize the fallacy of the concept sooner or later. The path to realization varies, but the time will come without fail. Then these people will ask themselves, "What has my life been for so far?" They would turn pale with consternation about the loss of all the time during which they were in the wrong. Those who apparently succeed in worldly possessions often realize this fact late in life. Those who were discouraged by illness or something usually realize it early.

Subsection 3: Significance of Human Lives

What is the significance of life, which all living creatures feel?

The conclusion that I reached is experience. It is to learn various feelings through various experiences. Among feelings, there are joy, sorrow, sympathy, anger, jealousy, fear, and more.

The most precious feeling is said to be that of love. There are many grades of love. Sometimes you think wrongly that you love somebody when you only like the person.

Many of you may think that parental love is pure and noble because the parents don't want the children to return the favor. However, in case you love your children in order to fulfill your own expectations, it is an egoistic love.

As long as human beings remain in the stage of egoistic love, there will be no progress in the global spiritual civilization. It is said that humans exist in order to learn the feeling of love that is directed to others without any condition or charge. You reincarnate, again and again, until you master this sort of love—changing countries, places, positions, sexes, you pile up experiences and learn. Just like actors in dramas, you experience a great many roles.

If you should wish that you were not born in your present circumstance but rather in a higher position like a king, I would say, "You already experienced a king. Your present life is supposed to be used for your experience as a king's servant or somebody who waits on others. Your soul has chosen your present environment for some reason." Some of you may think that you couldn't have chosen a miserable environment like this. Still, I must say, "You have chosen it by yourself, in order to become stronger against adversity and to comprehend deeper love." You should never be discouraged.

It is said that there is no coincidence; what happens to you happens with necessity. The same is true with the living environment. Namely, it is given as a place of trial, testing you if you are able to overcome the hardship. You also should overcome your disease, if you are sick. It is no time to be pessimistic.

Subsection 4: Purpose of Life

You cannot know exactly when you will die. Therefore, you are able to live easily. In childhood, you grow up with aid of parents or relatives. After required education, you may go to schools of higher grade, or you may begin to work. In adulthood, you fall in love with someone, form a connection, and get married. After the marriage, children are born, and the parents are kept busy attending to the baby. After the kids grow up, their own lives begin. Parents follow up on their children's lives for as long as possible. We repeat these things over generations and live our limited span of life. What is the purpose of our lives?

Many of you might have never thought of such a thing. Under the present conditions, many people are kept busy working to live every day. However, those who are suffering from incurable diseases might think, *What is my life?*

I previously wrote about the significance of human lives, but I would like to discuss now the purpose of human lives.

Some of you may say, "It's health." But health is not a purpose; it is a means to accomplish the purpose.

You may say, "It's to become as rich as possible." The reason why you say so must be because you believe that rich people are free from financial troubles and can get a perfect freedom. However, in the global civilization of today, you'll never get peace of mind even if you and your family become wealthy. That is because innumerous people are starving on this planet.

The earth can't be a stable planet as long as these poor people exist. There are so many poor people because the earth is infested with terrorism and other crimes. Several years ago, a war broke out, making a campaign of "war against terrorism." Among wars, this war is fought between an overwhelmingly military country and lesser powers.

Granting that you became wealthy, you couldn't be free from anxiety in the world, where you may be involved in a war or a dispute. Human beings are creatures that are unable to be fully glad alone while some people are starving or are committing suicide.

In the Roman era, Jesus Christ taught people, "Love thy neighbor." He said, "Take care of people around you," and "Keep on living sympathizing with each other." In the Roman era, there was war after war in order to expand territory. The Romans conquered the surrounding countries and gained trophies and tributes, bringing wealth to Rome. The aristocracy conducted political affairs through the Senatus and enjoyed graceful lives. The graceful lives of Romans, who were the conquerors, were supported by the sacrifice of the surrounding countries. Two thousand years have passed since the Roman empire flourished.

Unfortunately, nothing has changed. The desire to control the world has been continued by other countries after the Romans. War does not disappear. Even now, wars or disputes are being fought here and there on this planet. How long do we have to continue these destructive actions before we realize our foolishness?

Japan underwent a big defeat during World War II. But thanks to the Peace Constitution ("We permanently abandon military powers as means of settlement of international conflicts."), we have spent the time since then without any war. However, now that those who experienced the war have grown old, and the majority population is those who have no experience of war, the number of people who realize the virtue of the Peace Constitution is decreasing. There still are statesmen of power who have the ambition of leading their country profitably. Persons who have a personal desire to satisfy themselves, even by killing the other party, still exist. A world where egoism pushes its way is unstable and brings about destruction without fail. People build up civilizations, and then others destroy the whole thing. These repetitions are the history of this planet. It is about time we human beings awake. It is the time to realize that there is no ultimate personal happiness without happiness of the whole. It is the time to think about what you can do to help the happiness of the whole.

There is a great variety in people's personal ability. You ought to contribute to the world according to your ability. There is no rank among occupations. Can you say that people engaged in cleaning streets are inferior to politicians or ministers? How noble are the people who silently keep cleaning the streets, compared to the egoists who conduct politics, pursuing connections for money!

Politicians ought to do their best for the sake of public, making good use of their ability. As for school education, it is time to improve its contents. I would suggest that social services be incorporated into the curriculum to cultivate the spirit of serving others. You taste and experience the spirit of service through the practical exercise of that service.

Herein lies the purpose for which we are going to go on living in the twenty-first century. The rest depends on whether you put it into action.

Subsection 5: Suicide

The number of people who choose suicide should decrease if the purpose of their present lives is shown plainly. However, this has yet to happen. In Japan each year, more than thirty thousand people, who have healthy physical bodies, choose the path of suicide. From the viewpoint of sick people, they must think, *What a waste!* Rarely does a sick person commit suicide, being too pessimistic to stay alive. Recently, the elderly population increased, as have cases in which an elderly person takes care of another elderly person. Consequently, the caregiver tends to get exhausted and sick. Sometimes there are tragic incidents, such as the attendant killing the sick, or sometimes a double suicide takes place.

There is no good reason why such tragedies should happen considering that they were luckily born in the twenty-first century. Even one suicide must not occur. A society where suicides are permitted can never be normal. You could say that such a society is not a civilized society.

There are a variety of hardships facing the people who commit suicide. Their direct motive may be either that they reached a conclusion that there was no choice but to die, or that they did it in the spur of the moment. The most frequent motive of suicide is related to money. People are unable to pay the bills or to maintain the family. The currency that was invented to serve people is now a tool to deprive them of their lives. We ought to aim for a world where money does not exist because it is unnecessary.

There are some people who commit suicide because they have lost their love or are unable to marry that person. There are cases where some boys or girls commit suicide after being teased at school. Grown-ups are certainly responsible for suicides of under-ages. Both givers and receivers of teasing are victims of the present society, which is able to give the underaged neither a dream nor an aim.

In cases of grown-ups, the opportunities to overcome the hardships are available to each person. If you killed yourself, you would be regarded as having failed in overcoming the hardship. Then you would have to carry over your karma to your next life and do it over again. Consequently, you have spent your present life in vain.

You ought to learn the "mechanism of life" before you decide to commit suicide. All who wish to commit suicide are prejudiced that nothing is immortal; in other words, souls don't exist. In this connection, however, the truth is that souls do exist as immortal entities.

Please remind yourself that souls overlap physical bodies as far as living matters are concerned. Physical bodies get exhausted and perish sooner or later, because they are finite. Only a few people live for a hundred years. However, your soul, which is your real entity, survives the deaths of your physical bodies. Souls go to the other world from this world.

Some of you may think that these discussions have nothing to do with medicine. But I would dare say that these discussions must guide you to an enlightenment, which will reduce the extent of the stress you feel. Accordingly, these discussions should help you remain in better health.

As I discuss in more detail in the next chapter, this world consists of three dimensions, and the other world—that is, the spiritual world—consists of multiple dimensions, from the fourth dimension through the ninth. To what dimension of the spiritual world you go when you physically die depends on how you spend your life in this world. The grade of your mind— whether you lived egoistically or affectionately—will determine the dimension of the spiritual world to which you go. The reason why our souls and minds are invisible is because they are made of high-frequency waves. Physical bodies are made of the lowest frequency waves, and souls are made of higher frequency waves. Among souls, there are varieties of wave frequencies depending on the owner's mind. The higher the wave frequency, the higher the dimension of the spiritual world to which the soul belongs.

Subsection 6: Are We Actively Living or Passively Being Kept Alive?

Most of us think that we are living by our own ability, but is that really so? Do flowers in the field grow and flower by their own wills? Plants grow, flower, and yield seeds when the season comes even if they had no will. Everything in nature is like this; it is the cosmic providence, or the natural providence.

Recently, the global climate changed vigorously. The ice in the Arctic and Antarctic regions is melting, being caused by the globally warmer climate and bringing about rise of sea levels, sinking land, droughts, and floods. In the United States of America, hurricanes raged, and tornadoes took place in Japan. The frequency of their occurrence is increasing, and their ferocity is growing.

Atmospheric and ocean currents are also changing their movements vigorously, and something unusual is happening regarding the catching of fish. Following the rise of temperature of sea, coral reefs are dying. The number of species of plants and animals on the earth that are going to die out is increasing. Cessation of these phenomena is beyond the human power. Curtailing carbon dioxide is a contemporary global topic, but there are discrepancies between opinions of participating countries, and it is doubtful whether we will reach the goal. Even if we reach the goal, it is uncertain whether we can stop the fluctuations of nature. No living beings would survive if the sun should disappear. If daylight time were drastically shortened, plants wouldn't grow properly, resulting in shortage of food.

All of us simply expect the natural phenomena to keep occurring as they used to do, but there is no guarantee. Nobody is capable of foreseeing precisely what will happen in the future. When disaster actually happens, we should realize that the thought "We are living by our own ability" was a conceit and nothing but an illusion.

We ought to realize that we have been kept alive due to the great favor of nature. If you do so, you would become modest.

You possess your position and your property, but you shouldn't think you got them only by yourself. The same is true with your health. If you think that everything was a gift, you can't live greedily and egocentrically enjoying exclusive possession of them. Thinking that you are kept alive to receive all necessities, you would be free from dissatisfaction, discontent, anxieties, and complaints. In addition, you will be spontaneously grateful and able to say "Thank you" to anybody and anything. On your way to your future life, whatever may happen, you will overcome them and be calmly grateful in the end. Those who can do so are the genuine victors of life.

Comparing your fate with others, you might think, *How could I be grateful when I am so miserable?*

In my youth, I was able to get over a hardship while experiencing a similar circumstance. Frankly speaking, I asked myself, *Is my present agony the biggest among the people on the earth?* I realized that it was not; there were numerous people who were less lucky. I remember that I felt relieved, as if a dark cloud faded away.

Suicide is regarded as more sinful than murder. In cases of murders, there are causes of the conflict that are usually revealed by the murderer. In cases of suicides, only the will of the one who dies matters. It is a proof of lack of knowledge to choose suicide easily. You ought not to die in a state of ignorance. You ought to die after having learned something from this life.

Subsection 7: Post-mortem World

Some people confidently declare, "The post-mortem world does not exist because nobody can prove it, and nobody came back after death." I say that they are ignorant because there are records of thorough scientific studies on the post-mortem world performed in the eighteenth century through the beginning of the twentieth century, such as the famous studies of Emanuel Swedenborg and of Sir Arthur Conan Doyle. There are numerous examples where a living person communicated with a dead person, or where the soul of a dead person materialized.

In the eighteenth century, Emanuel Swedenborg performed a research study about the spiritual world. He visited the spiritual world repeatedly, leaving his physical body home in this world, and wrote a large number of books, such as *Arcana Coelestia* (Latin title meaning *Secrets of Heaven*) describing his experience during his visit. He was regarded at the time as a spiritualist or a scholar of psychics.

In 1920, the soul named Silver Birch entered the body of Morris Barbannel. Through Barbannel, Silver Birch gave messages concerning the spiritual world and the cosmic law for sixty years. If these studies had not been discontinued, the existence of the post-mortem world would have become common knowledge.

However, it appears that teaching people about the immortality of life was inconvenient for the power that intended to rule and control the whole world. That is because men of power found that the most effective means in order to rule people were to give fear to the people. The most typical fear is that of death. Death is fearful for most people; we want to live eternally if possible. It is because we think that everything ends with death. If you can believe firmly that souls with personalities survive physical deaths and can play active parts, then your fear toward death will shrink a great deal.

In the age of Japanese civil wars, men of power cut off and exposed to the public the heads of those who resisted the power in order to raise public fear and make people obey. The same was true in Europe; guillotines in the French Revolution created nothing but fear. The reason why the death penalty exists in contemporary society is also because nations attempt to stabilize society by threatening people with death.

As far as the ruling power is concerned, it is undesirable that the common people come to know the immortality of souls. Few people would fear death after they know that death is the start of journeys to the other world. It will be a hindrance for the rulers.

Under these circumstances, the studies, which were supposed to scientifically demonstrate the presence of a post-mortem world and were going to guide human beings to a brilliant dawn, were forcefully stopped.

Subsection 8: To Overcome Fears

Let's think about where fear generally comes from.

In the first place, there is a fear concerning daily lives. Fear of job loss, unstable or insufficient income, lack of food or shelter, and the inability to afford children's education and health—all these fears are connected with money.

There are mental fears, too: not being allowed to join a social circle, not being treated equally, getting teased, not being helped, having no guidance. There are fears of being left alone, being looked down upon, and being ignored.

Ultimately, there is a fear of being threatened with loss of life. The global confusion of swine influenza, which arose in 2009, was such a cause of fear. There also is the risk of being assassinated when you face a big power for the sake of justice. However vicious a law may be, unless you obey it, the worst penalty is to be sentenced to death. Not only must you die, but also your beloved family may be involved.

Unless you get rid of fears, you will be unable to advance.

In the United States, many people keep pistols or rifles in their homes for self-defense. There are some districts in the United States where you can't walk around due to a danger of being shot by those weapons—which are being used not for self-defense but for attacking somebody else. This situation is a problem of individuals, but you can apply the story to nations. Today, the world takes a small step toward the reduction and abolition of nuclear armaments. Why can't they part with nuclear weapons completely?

Iran and North Korea are criticized by nuclear powers for not stopping their development of nuclear weapons. India and Pakistan obtained nuclear devices and joined the nuclear powers—the United States, Russia, Great Britain, China, France, and Israel. The global world is divided into nuclear powers and nonnuclear powers. Nuclear powers won't part with the weapons, and nonnuclear nations plan to obtain the weapons. Just like people keeping guns in their homes, the nations want to revenge in case they are attacked with nuclear weapons, or they believe that they won't be attacked if they were equipped with the weapons. They misunderstand and believe that to have nuclear devices is to protect their own countries. The concept of preemptive attack is to beat the enemy before you are beaten.

In the background of the nuclear conflict are anxieties and fears of being attacked by the enemy. If no one had nuclear weapons, nobody would need to be worried about nuclear attack.

As long as human beings are incapable of overcoming fears, they will keep being incapable of abolishing nuclear weapons. If the weapons are developed in more nations, the risk of their usage would be higher.

Now is the time when the global human beings must give full play to their wisdom.

As stated above, unless each person conquers the fear of death, it is inevitable that nations, which are a collective of individuals, are influenced by fears of the enforcement of policies. Fears that arise in the course of life should be extinguished by knowing the significance of human lives.

Your fear for your death, the most serious of all, could be made less so by realizing the mechanism and mystery of life. Knowing that your soul is real and that you will survive the physical body's death, you won't be desperate or anxious.

CHAPTER 5:
Prospects for the Future

Subsection 1: Toward an Optimistic World

Following the economical crisis that originated in the United States in 2008, enterprises have frequently declared bankruptcy, the number of unemployed rapidly increased in all countries, and the extent of social confusion deepened. In Afghanistan and Iraq, disputes and terrorism never cease.

Similar conditions are also seen in Japan. Incomprehensible and impulsive murders occur frequently. Unemployed people are anywhere, and employed people's incomes go down. Uneasiness is amplified, and cities are crowded by people who have lost their hopes.

Some people declare, "It is a providential rule of nature that the strong gets selected, leaving the weak behind." They may say, "The expansion of earning differentials are in accordance with the natural law." Certainly in the animal kingdom, it may be applied. However, human beings are equipped with intelligence. There is no reason whatsoever why we should be like animals.

We ought to aim for an unbiased society, where we think of the whole society, not only of ourselves or our families. We should think of harmony with the people around us, take care of someone in need, and more. A society where only some people are well paid is not right.

It is said that the global society is entering a new stage. Whether or not you believe the saying, I am one of those who believe in the "grand change" of the earth. Needless to say, I think the earth will turn to a society of hope.

As I have said so many times, the society where competitive spirits are stirred up, people are driven by money, and large earning differentials are approved is going to vanish sooner or later. It is going to change into a society where people have composure, sympathy to each other, and mental peace.

Subsection 2: Problems That the Earth Must Conquer

As I have already stated, the force that drives humans is money. Most activities are in pursuit of money. Now, money has become a sort of faith; it even controls human life. People sometimes take a life for money or commit suicide because of money. To a person who thinks that he cannot live without money, money is an entity just like God—or even more precious than God.

We must extinguish this faith toward money.

What kind of movement will there be if we should succeed in extinguishing money from this world? The global civilization has been built up by competition. Everybody thinks it is a matter of course that human beings compete with each other, and the competing spirit has contributed to the development of civilization and human society.

What would happen if we eliminate the competing spirit? Would every progress and development cease?

Many people believe that nobody would voluntarily work, and social efficacy would go down in a society where there is no competition and everybody is treated equally. But would it be really so? Competitions give birth to earning differentials. Winners are well paid, take higher positions, and can live comfortably. Losers are compelled to live miserably. This is the earthly rule.

However, is this the ideal society? In order to be a winner, extraordinary efforts and talents are required. If you injure your health a great deal, you would be a loser instantaneously. Losers would produce friction against winners, bringing about social uneasiness. Dissatisfied lives may drive a loser to commit a crime. Crimes will never cease in societies where there are large earning differentials.

In competitive societies, the dream of social peace will never come true because losers will always be created by the competitions.

In our future society, the competitive principle will not work. Some people may be afraid that nobody will be willing to work without competition. However, in the future, the motive to work will be quite different.

Now, what do you think will be the motive to work in a society where neither money nor positions exist?

In those societies, it is an utmost joy to work for others, to serve others, and to do something for the sake of others. The joy of serving others is great, and there will be nothing else needed as a purpose of work. The joy of displaying one's ability cannot be replaced by anything.

Unfortunately, such a society does not exist on this planet—yet.

The feature of the earth today is that most people are working, feeling pains, exhausting their nerves, and being tortured in order to fulfill assigned tasks.

Subsection 3: Warless World

Why are we unable to cease wars?

One of the causes is because money is the purpose of life for some people, and therefore they cannot change the mechanism of competition to attain a better purpose.

We need to aim for a society where we equally share everything, not scramble for competition. We have come to our current limit; there will be neither mental evolution nor global development while egoism continues to dominate.

There are starving people who have nothing to eat today, while wealthy people enjoy their lives as they choose. There are rich and poor nations, and so troubles and disputes won't disappear. International wars break out due to plunders and exploitations. A powerful nation carries on a war in order to take away resources to satisfy their own limitless desire. The nation who has been bolstered by a war makes efforts to increase armaments.

Another cause of war is the fear of being killed by others. Nations think that they ought to have armaments to kill the enemy before they get killed themselves. This is a vicious circle. What should we do to overcome the fear of death? The answer is that we need to learn the mechanism of life and the cosmic law to be enlightened. When human beings have overcome the fear of death, the global world will completely change. World peace can come true without weapons or armaments.

What would happen if you negotiated with another country of incompatible interest with no weapons or armaments? Many of you may think that you couldn't help obeying the opponent, who would threaten you with violence. However, such an idea comes from people who cannot throw away their egoism and desires for exclusive possession and conquest. When we have mastered the spirit of sharing everything, the results would entirely differ. Negotiate thoroughly and concede as much as possible.

What would happen if the opponent is unreasonable and tries to continue its egoism with its military power? The opponent may resort to war. However, if we have overcome the fear of death already, if we have full knowledge of the significance and purpose of human lives, and if we are in a situation where it is unnecessary to survive by killing the opponent, we won't fight, accepting death and being good losers.

Everything depends on whether the whole nation, especially the politicians, are able to conceive such a mental state. If you comprehend the cosmic providence and the law of karma, which I'm going to explain in the next subsections, you would be more easily able to refrain from fighting.

How many more years would it take for the global world to throw weapons away and abolish wars? However time-consuming it may be, the time must come without fail. If it should fail to come, nuclear wars will cover the earth, human beings will die out, and this planet will die, too.

Subsection 4: Toward a Cosmic Age

Although we live in the third dimensional world, the universe is composed of multiple dimensional worlds. The global science has not elucidated the structure of the universe satisfactorily, yet. Although the farthest corner of the Milky Way is far beyond eyeshot, when we try to imagine the size of the cosmos, which is described in billions of light-years, we are surprised by its hugeness.

The solar system is said to have eight planets, but in fact twelve planets exist according to the late Mr. Shinji Takahashi, one of the greatest human beings, whose physical body lived in Japan for forty-nine years (1927–1976). He also says that the ancestor of the global human beings came from Andromeda nebula as a group of sixty million people riding on six thousand cigar-shaped space ships three hundred and sixty-five million years ago. They landed on African continent and created a harmonized community. The leader of that group created the global divine world after his physical death. His soul named himself El Ranty, who reincarnated as Shinji Takahashi. He also declared in 1990 through Ryuho Ohkawa that none of Yahveh, Jehovah, and Allah is the Creator although there is a traditional faith that they are. He declares that the above three names are the other names of El Ranty. In other words, his declaration is an authentication of the fact that Christianity, Judaism, and Islam are religions of one same great entity; El Ranty. According to Shinji Takahashi, the purpose of his life in the twentieth century was to save the global world from its terminal crisis uniting the three religions; Christianity, Judaism, and Islam, notifying the believers of the religions of the fact that each of Jehovah, Yahveh, and Allah is just another name of El Ranty. He still also says that

Darwinism is not relevant. In his opinion, human beings were created by the Creator *per se* and *de novo*. The same is true with other beings; animals, plants, and minerals although evolution did take place within a species, for example, horses a million years ago were much smaller in size than they are, today. He also points out as evidence of irrelevancy of Darwinism the absence of intermediaries between plural species, for example, monkey and human being.

It is said that in the Milky Way there are two hundred billion stars, on most of which life exists. It is also said that there are two hundred billion galaxies in the cosmos. It is still also said that numerous other cosmos exist forming a shape of a human body as a whole, supporting the relevancy of the legend that tells you that God created a macrocosm in resemblance of His own shape, according to Mr. Ryuho Ohkawa, also one of the greatest human entities born in Tokushima, Japan in 1956, who also says that this cosmos of ours occupies the right eye of the macrocosm. When we hear that numerous cosmos exist, the hugeness is beyond our capacity of comprehension. Besides, there also are worlds of different dimensions, including the post-mortem world. There also seems to be a world where the past and the future simultaneously exist with the present, which is beyond our imagination. In such a world, it is possible to go back to the past, to several thousand years ago, and one can also go to the future.

The visiting aliens seem to have advanced several thousand years ahead of us, and they are anxious about us because we are retarded in mental evolution. They are waiting for the time when human beings graduate from the barbarism of attacking others and cease wars. Then they will show up publicly, with dignity.

Considering this, this is not a time when we should keep fighting on the earth, which is infinitesimally small compared to the hugeness of the macrocosm. It is the time to learn from those who are advanced and to pay attention to the macrocosm.

Subsection 5: Cosmic Law

In the vast universe, including the earth, solemn laws exist.

You can call the entity that has created the macrocosm and that controls it perfectly God. You can also call the entity the Great Divine Spirit. Although there are various names for it, you should know that you owe the Great Wisdom for the smooth running of the macrocosm.

In accordance with the fact that the Great Wisdom is not chaotic, there exists a cosmic law that cannot be changed or altered by anybody. We call it dharma, and it is not a man-made law.

At this point I would like to explain the cosmic law. You may have heard the phrase, "Everything transmigrates." It is said that these words are the proverb that was given by Herakleitos around 500 BC, but the truth is not clear. To transmigrate means not to stay or stop. Everything in the universe is ceaselessly changing. The changes direct us toward advancements. No stagnation is allowed. Accordingly, it is said that human lives also undergo metempsychosis or vicissitudes—reincarnation. In other words, human lives repeatedly go and return from this world to another world; we are reborn after we die.

Souls who continue their training on earth are born. As a matter of course, they often change countries, places, and times. If a soul can get out of the ring of reincarnation, it is not necessary for the soul to receive training. In other words, the soul has graduated from earthly training.

Among the laws controlling the universe, there is the law of causality. It is also called the law of karma. The law tells you, "You must harvest what you have seeded." It means that what you have done to somebody will come back to you without fail. Suppose a person cheated somebody else, and the one who was cheated therefore suffered and died. The cheater has given himself a karma and will be cheated and will suffer sometime in the future.

Such phenomena cannot always be liquidated during one life span. Sometimes you atone for the karma you made in your previous life. Generally speaking, we have no memory of our previous lives because the memory gets erased when we are born in this world. It's because it is more convenient for the spiritual growth. Rarely does the erased memory revive.

Suppose there is an unreasonable relationship, and a person says, "Why am I treated like this while I am sincerely serving my love?" You couldn't solve the mystery within the span of your present life. However, it would be apparent that you are atoning for your karma if you take your previous life into consideration.

Similar circumstances are seen in cases of illnesses. Especially in cases of stiffness of hands and feet, the cause of illness often originates in previous lives. If you had died while suffering from a horrible mortification, the karma appears as an illness.

Don't be pessimistic because your karma will vanish sooner or later. However painful it may be, it will fade away as you endure, and you will feel gratitude for the opportunity that allows you to atone for your karma, which you have forgotten.

There also is good karma. Some people are always fortunate, and others may think, *Why is he so lucky all the time?* It is because his karma is showing up. In case you have given and distributed your love to others in your previous lives, the return will visit in your present life.

Regardless of others, your good deeds will come back to you without fail.

What would you do if you killed a stranger, running over him by your car while driving under the influence of liquor? It is so troublesome to make up for the accident. You may need to take care of the bereaved family till you die. If you enter a jail, you would lose your social credit and position. The reparation might be too heavy for you. You think about this and that. Looking around, you see nobody. You think that you could make escape unnoticed.

People are tested at such a time. Once you escape, you take a big hit in karma. It does not matter whether the police find out about your crime or whether you make your escape. That is merely a matter of this world. One who performs a terrible action will have the action returned to him in the next life. Sometimes, persons of no relationship are killed by a phantom. Although these incidents should never happen, here the law of karma is acting. Those who were killed abruptly had a debt in their previous lives. Males who mistreated females in previous lives will be mistreated by the opposite sex in this life. Thus, thanks to the law of karma, you can learn from your previous failures.

In order to get rid of the law of karma, you should forgive other people thoroughly. You could graduate from the law if you forgive your opponent without accusing or confronting him, however unreasonable he may be.

Applying this theory to international affairs, you would reach a conclusion that you should never respond with war to your opponent, even if the opponent should kill you. Because lives are immortal, you would be reborn on a warless, peaceful planet even if you get killed and leave this world. You won't need to worry at all; you can go on dying gladly.

Unfortunately, one thousand more years might be necessary for the contemporary world to attain such a mental state.

Subsection 6: New Way of Life

It seems to me that the reason why we keep repeating struggling is because human beings don't have trustworthy dreams or aims in their lives. We understand our lives as short time spans, deny invisible entities, and incorrectly believe that nothing but visible things exist. Consequently, we overlook extremely important points. Our way of living would change a great deal if we were able to recognize that our souls exist permanently.

We would also become unable to continue a foolish war against another nation if we changed our purpose of life from the low-dimensional idea of "earning money through competition" to a grand dream of learning the truth from the universe. We would realize that it is time to stop arguing over trifles when we could visit other planets that are highly civilized.

There are innumerous things that we ought to learn and rejoice. We waste our time being attached to insignificant things merely because we are ignorant about things of higher importance. It is said that the earth does not stay at the present level, but it will jump up soon. That means that we would be unable to stay on the earth unless we raise our own levels.

Now, what is the new way of living in the cosmic age? There are a number of religions on the earth. Although there are inter-religious debates, why do people need religions? The answer is because people cannot trust themselves and want to rely upon someone who may help and guide them.

The majority of people pray to God or Buddha for their recoveries when they are sick. But however long they may pray, God does not help, and the results don't change. Would an illness be cured by praying at home?

God quietly helps those who make efforts to live voluntarily and take actions while trusting their own abilities. Human beings are equipped with a similar power as God; we are merely incapable of realizing it. However, it is not that everybody can display an infinite power. All you do is to try as much as you can and leave the rest to the heaven. Then you will be grateful for the result no matter what it is. This is what I mean by living positively.

To believe in the wisdom that unifies the universe and to join a religious organization are quite different. Religions are man-made. Jesus and Mohammed taught how to live but made no organizations. In the age to come, there will be neither religions nor religious organizations.

Subsection 7: Self-Consciousness of Global Human Beings

I would like to summarize what I have stated up to here.

I have a sincere wish to offer a novel method of healing diseases that used to be incurable so that patients can resume complete health. I also have a desire that the healthy people who used to be patients will spend the rest of their lives with enlightenment.

Those who have read this book must have realized that our lives are not single ones but a part of eternity. This is a concept concerning time. From the viewpoint of space, our earth is a tiny object in the great big universe. In addition, our earth is just one of trillions of planets where highly civilized beings live.

Both you and I were born on a same planet. We were not born aimlessly or coincidentally. We were born with a certain plan, although we do not remember the plan at all. There is a reason for the birth of every person: to make your soul spiritually grow up and to guide the earth to a peaceful, harmonized, and tranquil world. You liquidate the karma of your previous life performing your mission.

Before long, the human beings will reach the cosmic age. The time will come when we look to extraterrestrial beings for assistance.

What we Japanese are supposed to do in the near future is to spread our Peace Constitution to the world; we must make it a global constitution. We ought to make a weaponless world, and especially remove nuclear weapons.

In the second place, we need to promote the harmonization of earning differentials. Richer nations aid poor nations gratis. Each nation should be equally rich and be released from poverty and famine.

In conclusion, unless you know the truth of universe, you tend to spend your lives for third-dimensional matters. The value of knowing and practicing the cosmic law cannot be replaced by anything.

EPILOGUE

I have published this book in order to offer good news to those who are suffering from incurable diseases and who are perplexed by difficulty of curing the disease in spite of treatment.

I was struck with an idea that led me to the ultimate method as I spent every day keeping in mind the question, "What is a radical cure for allergic diseases?"

I promptly tested the idea on patients after informed consent. Results of the test were superb. Every patient showed improvement. I tried to publish my article in an authoritative journal, but for unknown reasons, I received no response. I also met an authoritative scholar of immunology who recognized and agreed with my idea first, but later he did nothing for its popularization. It became apparent to me what kind of trend was leading the global as well as Japanese immunological societies.

Although an effective treatment has been discovered, it wouldn't spread into the world. During these years, I kept practicing the method in my own medical clinic and obtained a number of clinical cases. As a last resort, I chose to publicize the method through this book.

There is nothing else I expect but that my method of healing incurable diseases will spread into the whole world, and patients will be saved. If my dream comes true, I would be able to contribute to the world through medicine, which I have learned and practiced for a lifetime.

Frankly speaking, my motivation of getting this book published is an extremely noble one. I have literally no desire for fame, honor, or money. All I want is to save those who suffer from currently incurable diseases.

Hopefully, the term 'currently' shall change to 'previously' shortly. The more shortly, the better. It's up to you how shortly it'll change, namely, it's up to how firmly you trust my words. God bless you!

ACKNOWLEDGMENTS

I am grateful to a friend of mine, Mr. Masashi Gotoh, for writing a major part of the Japanese manuscript, which I translated into English and added my own information.

I am also grateful to Mr. Ryuho Ohkawa and the late Mr. Shinji Takahashi, who gave us information about the spiritual world as well as the macrocosm.

KIMIHIKO OKAZAKI graduated from Kyoto University Faculty of Medicine in 1959 and conducted medical chemical research for twenty-one years, during which time he made achievements such as discoveries of 'A novel coenzyme in Baker's yeast' and 'Initiator of rat liver regeneration'. He has specialized in internal medicine since 1981 and is running a private clinic in Kyoto since 1989.